AI

HEALTHCARE

Intelligent Insights: Transforming Healthcare with AI-Driven Diagnostics

Erkan YILDIRIM

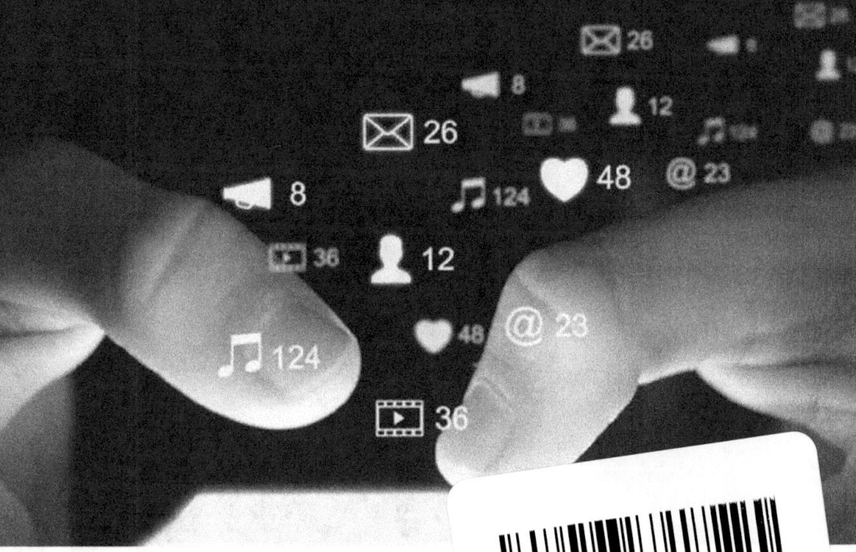

Chapter 1: Introduction to AI in Healthcare

The Evolution of Healthcare Technology

The evolution of healthcare technology has been a remarkable journey, marked by continuous innovation and the integration of advanced tools that have transformed patient care. Historically, healthcare relied heavily on manual processes and rudimentary tools for diagnostics and treatment. The introduction of computers in the late 20th century began to change this landscape, enabling healthcare professionals to store and analyze patient data more efficiently. As technology progressed, the advent of electronic health records (EHRs) became a cornerstone for modern healthcare, facilitating better communication among providers and streamlining patient management.

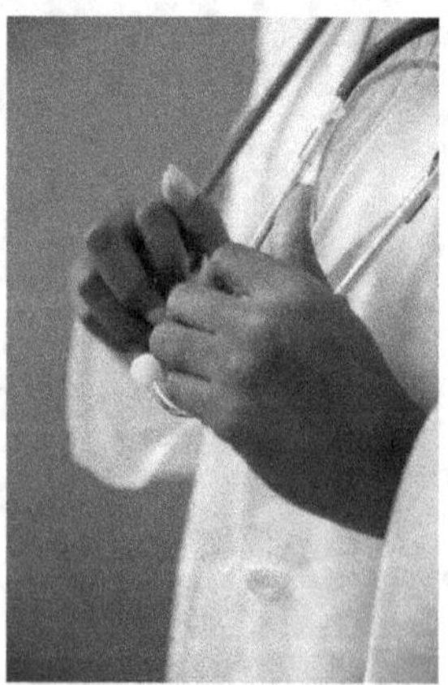

With the turn of the century, the evolution of technology accelerated, particularly with the rise of the internet and mobile devices. This shift allowed for more accessible healthcare information and telemedicine solutions, which became especially vital during the COVID-19 pandemic. The ability to conduct remote consultations not only minimized the risk of virus transmission but also highlighted the importance of integrating technology into everyday healthcare practices. As healthcare systems adapted to these changes, the demand for AI-driven diagnostic tools and predictive analytics surged, paving the way for more personalized approaches to patient care.

The incorporation of artificial intelligence into healthcare has revolutionized diagnostic capabilities. AI technologies can analyze vast amounts of data at unprecedented speeds, identifying patterns and anomalies that may elude human observation. In medical imaging, for instance, AI algorithms enhance image analysis, improving the accuracy of diagnostics in radiology and pathology. This has significant implications for early disease detection and treatment planning, allowing healthcare professionals to make more informed decisions based on data-driven insights.

Furthermore, AI's potential in personalized medicine cannot be overstated. By leveraging genetic information and patient history, AI systems can help tailor treatment plans to individual patients, enhancing efficacy and minimizing adverse effects. This transition from a one-size-fits-all approach to personalized therapies represents a significant shift in how healthcare is delivered. Additionally, AI facilitates drug discovery and development, expediting the identification of potential therapeutic candidates and reducing the time and cost associated with bringing new drugs to market.

As we look to the future, the implications of AI in mental health monitoring and support also warrant attention. AI-driven platforms can provide continuous assessment and real-time feedback, enabling healthcare providers to intervene more effectively. The evolution of healthcare technology is not merely about the tools themselves but also about how these innovations can enhance the overall patient experience. As healthcare professionals, researchers, and technologists collaborate, the integration of AI into healthcare systems promises to deliver more efficient, effective, and personalized care, ultimately improving outcomes for patients worldwide.

Overview of AI and Its Applications

Artificial Intelligence (AI) has emerged as a transformative technology across various sectors, particularly in healthcare. Defined as the simulation of human intelligence processes by machines, AI encompasses a range of techniques including machine learning, natural language processing, and neural networks. These technologies enable systems to analyze vast amounts of data, learn from it, and make predictions or decisions based on that information. In healthcare, AI's ability to process and interpret complex datasets—such as clinical records, medical images, and genomic information—offers unprecedented opportunities for improving patient outcomes and streamlining medical workflows.

One of the most significant applications of AI in healthcare is in diagnostic tools. AI-driven diagnostic systems leverage algorithms to analyze medical images, identify patterns, and assist clinicians in making accurate diagnoses. For instance, AI has shown promise in detecting conditions such as cancer through radiological images, where it can outperform traditional methods in terms of speed and accuracy. Moreover, these tools can help reduce the burden on radiologists, allowing them to focus on more complex cases and improving overall efficiency in diagnostic processes.

Personalized medicine is another area where AI is making substantial strides. By analyzing patient data, including genetic information and lifestyle factors, AI systems can tailor treatment plans to individual patients, enhancing the effectiveness of therapies while minimizing side effects. This approach not only improves patient satisfaction but also optimizes resource allocation within healthcare systems. As more data becomes available, the potential for AI to refine and personalize treatment protocols continues to grow, paving the way for a more targeted approach to healthcare.

In addition to diagnostics and personalized medicine, AI plays a critical role in predictive analytics for patient care. By examining historical patient data, AI algorithms can identify trends and predict potential health issues before they arise. This proactive approach allows healthcare providers to intervene early, manage chronic conditions more effectively, and reduce hospital admissions. Furthermore, AI's applications extend to drug discovery and development, where it accelerates the identification of potential therapeutic compounds and streamlines clinical trials, significantly reducing the time and cost involved in bringing new medications to market.

AI-enhanced telemedicine solutions are also revolutionizing patient care, especially in the context of increasing demand for remote healthcare services. Through AI-driven platforms, healthcare providers can offer real-time consultations, monitor patient health remotely, and deliver personalized health interventions. Additionally, AI is being utilized in mental health monitoring and support, where it can analyze patient interactions and provide insights into mental well-being. This integration of AI not only enhances the accessibility of healthcare services but also ensures that patients receive timely and relevant support, further underscoring the vast potential of AI in transforming the healthcare landscape.

Chapter 2: AI-Driven Diagnostic Tools

Types of AI Diagnostic Tools

AI diagnostic tools can be categorized into several distinct types, each serving specific functions that enhance the accuracy and efficiency of healthcare delivery. One prominent category is medical imaging analysis tools, which utilize deep learning algorithms to interpret complex imaging data from modalities such as X-rays, MRIs, and CT scans. These tools can identify anomalies, assist in early diagnosis of conditions like cancer, and streamline radiology workflows, allowing healthcare professionals to focus on patient care rather than time-consuming image analysis.

Another vital category includes predictive analytics tools, which leverage vast datasets to forecast patient outcomes and disease progression. By analyzing historical patient data, these tools can identify risk factors and predict potential complications, enabling healthcare providers to implement preventive measures tailored to individual patients. This personalized approach is particularly valuable in managing chronic diseases, where timely interventions can significantly improve patient quality of life and reduce healthcare costs.

AI-driven decision support systems represent a third type of diagnostic tool, which aids clinicians in making informed treatment choices. These systems integrate patient data, evidence-based guidelines, and clinical pathways to provide recommendations that align with the latest research. By reducing cognitive load and supporting clinical reasoning, these tools enhance the decision-making process, ultimately leading to improved patient outcomes and more efficient use of healthcare resources.

Telemedicine solutions enhanced by AI also play a crucial role in modern diagnostics, particularly in rural and underserved areas where access to specialty care may be limited. AI algorithms can analyze patient data collected through remote monitoring devices and provide real-time feedback to both patients and healthcare providers. This not only facilitates timely interventions but also empowers patients to take an active role in their health management, fostering a more collaborative healthcare environment.

Lastly, AI's application in mental health monitoring and support tools is increasingly recognized as essential. These tools employ natural language processing and machine learning to analyze patient interactions, assess emotional states, and provide tailored interventions. By identifying patterns in patient behavior and sentiment, these tools enable clinicians to deliver personalized mental health care, enhancing treatment efficacy and supporting patients through their recovery journeys. Collectively, these diverse AI diagnostic tools represent a transformative force in healthcare, paving the way for more accurate, efficient, and personalized patient care.

Benefits of AI in Diagnostics

The integration of artificial intelligence (AI) into healthcare diagnostics presents transformative benefits that significantly enhance the accuracy and efficiency of medical practices. One of the foremost advantages is the ability of AI-driven diagnostic tools to analyze vast amounts of data rapidly. Traditional diagnostic methods often involve time-consuming processes that can lead to delays in treatment. In contrast, AI algorithms can process complex datasets, including medical histories, lab results, and imaging data, in a fraction of the time. This swift analysis facilitates quicker decision-making and enables healthcare professionals to provide timely and effective interventions, ultimately improving patient outcomes.

AI's capacity for pattern recognition is another pivotal benefit in diagnostics. Machine learning algorithms excel at identifying subtle patterns in medical images, which may be overlooked by the human eye. In fields such as radiology and pathology, AI-enhanced imaging analysis can detect early signs of diseases like cancer, allowing for earlier interventions that can significantly improve survival rates. This capability not only augments the diagnostic accuracy but also helps in reducing the workload on healthcare professionals, enabling them to focus on more complex cases that require human expertise.

Personalized medicine is another area where AI demonstrates substantial benefits. By leveraging data from various sources, including genetic information and lifestyle factors, AI can assist in tailoring treatment plans to individual patients. This level of customization ensures that therapies are more effective and minimizes the trial-and-error approach often associated with traditional medicine. As a result, patients receive treatments that are specifically designed for their unique health profiles, enhancing the overall efficacy of care and improving their quality of life.

Furthermore, predictive analytics powered by AI plays a crucial role in patient care management. By analyzing historical data and trends, AI algorithms can forecast potential health issues before they arise, allowing for proactive measures to be taken. This predictive capability is particularly beneficial in managing chronic diseases, where early interventions can prevent complications and reduce hospitalizations. Healthcare administrators can also leverage these insights for resource allocation and strategic planning, ensuring that care facilities are well-equipped to meet the future demands of patient populations.

Lastly, AI's contributions extend to mental health monitoring and support, an area that has traditionally been challenging to address due to the subjective nature of diagnoses. AI-driven tools can analyze behavioral data and assess changes in mental health conditions, providing clinicians with valuable insights into their patients' well-being. Telemedicine solutions enhanced by AI further facilitate remote monitoring and support, making mental health resources more accessible. By combining these technological advancements, healthcare systems can offer comprehensive care that addresses both physical and mental health, ultimately leading to a more holistic approach to patient wellness.

Case Studies of Successful Implementations

Case studies of successful implementations of AI-driven diagnostics in healthcare illustrate the transformative potential of these technologies across various medical domains. One notable example is the integration of AI in radiology, where a leading hospital adopted an AI-powered imaging analysis tool to enhance the detection of lung cancer. This tool utilized deep learning algorithms to analyze thousands of chest X-rays and CT scans, allowing radiologists to identify malignancies with improved accuracy and speed. The implementation led to a 30% increase in the early detection rates of lung cancer, significantly impacting patient outcomes and underscoring the importance of AI in medical imaging analysis.

In the realm of personalized medicine, a healthcare organization implemented an AI-driven platform that analyzes genetic data alongside electronic health records to tailor treatment plans for cancer patients. By leveraging machine learning algorithms, the platform identified specific genetic mutations and correlated them with treatment responses observed in similar patient cohorts. This approach enabled oncologists to recommend targeted therapies, resulting in a notable improvement in treatment efficacy and a reduction in adverse effects. The success of this implementation emphasizes the role of AI in enhancing personalized treatment strategies.

AI-based predictive analytics is transforming patient care management in chronic disease populations. A case study from a large urban hospital demonstrated the implementation of an AI system designed to predict hospital readmissions for heart failure patients. By analyzing a multitude of factors, including previous admissions, socio-economic status, and clinical indicators, the AI model accurately predicted which patients were at highest risk of readmission. This insight allowed healthcare teams to intervene proactively with tailored discharge planning and follow-up care, leading to a marked decrease in readmission rates and associated healthcare costs.

Another compelling case is the deployment of AI-enhanced telemedicine solutions during the COVID-19 pandemic. A telehealth platform incorporated AI algorithms to triage patients based on their symptoms and medical history, directing them to appropriate care pathways. This innovation not only streamlined patient management but also ensured that healthcare providers could focus their efforts on patients with the most urgent needs. The rapid adoption of this technology highlighted the agility of healthcare systems and the potential for AI to improve access to care, particularly in times of crisis.

AI's role in drug discovery and development has also seen promising outcomes. A pharmaceutical company utilized AI algorithms to identify potential drug candidates for a rare disease. By sifting through vast datasets of molecular structures and biological interactions, the AI system accelerated the identification of compounds that could be effective in treating the condition. This case study demonstrated how AI can reduce the time and cost associated with drug development while increasing the likelihood of successful outcomes, showcasing its potential to revolutionize the pharmaceutical industry.

Chapter 3: Personalized Medicine Through AI

Understanding Personalized Medicine

Personalized medicine represents a revolutionary shift in healthcare, moving away from the traditional one-size-fits-all approach to a more tailored strategy that considers individual variability in genes, environment, and lifestyle. This paradigm shift is largely fueled by advancements in technology, notably artificial intelligence (AI), which enables healthcare providers to analyze vast amounts of data and derive insights that were previously unattainable. By leveraging AI-driven diagnostic tools, medical professionals can generate more precise diagnoses and treatment plans that cater specifically to the unique characteristics of each patient.

A fundamental aspect of personalized medicine is the integration of genomic information into clinical practice. With the ability to sequence genomes rapidly and cost-effectively, physicians can now identify genetic markers that influence a patient's response to various treatments. AI algorithms enhance this process by analyzing genomic data alongside other health metrics, allowing for a comprehensive understanding of a patient's health profile. This integration is particularly beneficial in areas such as oncology, where targeted therapies can be developed based on the specific mutations present in a patient's tumor.

In addition to genomic data, personalized medicine also considers a patient's medical history, lifestyle choices, and environmental factors. AI-driven predictive analytics play a crucial role in this context, enabling healthcare providers to forecast potential health outcomes based on a holistic view of the patient. By using machine learning models trained on extensive datasets, clinicians can identify risk factors and intervene early, potentially improving patient outcomes and reducing healthcare costs. This proactive approach not only enhances the quality of care but also empowers patients to take an active role in managing their health.

Moreover, the role of AI in medical imaging analysis cannot be understated. Advanced imaging techniques, combined with AI algorithms, facilitate the identification of abnormalities that may be missed by the human eye. These AI-enhanced solutions provide more accurate and timely diagnoses, which are essential for effective treatment planning. For instance, in radiology, machine learning models can analyze thousands of images to detect signs of diseases, such as cancer, at stages when they are most treatable. This capability underscores the importance of collaboration between physicians and data scientists in developing tools that further enhance personalized care.

Lastly, as telemedicine continues to gain traction, AI is transforming the way healthcare is delivered remotely. AI-driven platforms can monitor patients' health in real time, providing insights that help in managing chronic conditions and mental health issues. These systems analyze data from wearable devices and mobile applications, allowing healthcare providers to adjust treatment plans based on real-world evidence. By fostering a continuous connection between patients and providers, AI-enhanced telemedicine solutions not only improve access to care but also ensure that treatments remain aligned with the evolving needs of patients. Through personalized medicine, empowered by AI, the future of healthcare promises to be more effective, efficient, and patient-centered.

Role of AI in Tailoring Treatments

The role of artificial intelligence in tailoring treatments has emerged as a transformative force in healthcare, allowing for a more personalized approach to patient care. Traditional treatment methods often rely on generalized protocols that may not account for individual patient differences. However, AI algorithms can analyze vast datasets, including genetic information, medical histories, and lifestyle factors, to identify the most effective treatment options for specific patient populations. This capability enables healthcare professionals to move beyond a one-size-fits-all model and embrace a more nuanced understanding of patient needs.

AI-driven diagnostic tools play a crucial role in this process by providing real-time insights that inform treatment decisions. For instance, machine learning algorithms can analyze medical imaging data to detect anomalies that may not be visible to the human eye. By integrating these findings with patient-specific data, healthcare providers can develop tailored treatment plans that address the unique characteristics of each patient's condition. This approach not only enhances the accuracy of diagnoses but also optimizes the selection of interventions, ultimately leading to improved outcomes.

Personalized medicine through AI is particularly evident in oncology, where treatments can be customized based on the genetic makeup of both the patient and the tumor. AI technologies can process genomic data to identify mutations and other biomarkers that influence how a patient might respond to certain therapies. As a result, oncologists can select targeted therapies that are more likely to be effective, thus reducing the trial-and-error approach often associated with cancer treatment. This shift not only increases the likelihood of successful outcomes but also minimizes unnecessary side effects from ineffective treatments.

Predictive analytics plays a vital role in patient care by anticipating potential complications and adjusting treatment plans accordingly. AI systems can analyze patterns in patient data to predict disease progression and identify those at risk for adverse events. By harnessing this predictive capability, healthcare teams can implement preventive measures or adjust treatments proactively, thereby enhancing patient safety and optimizing resource allocation within healthcare settings. This proactive approach is particularly valuable in chronic disease management, where timely interventions can significantly alter disease trajectories.

The integration of AI in telemedicine solutions further underscores its role in tailoring treatments. Virtual consultations powered by AI can help healthcare providers assess patient conditions remotely, allowing for continuous monitoring and timely adjustments to treatment plans. For patients with mental health conditions, AI-enhanced tools can offer real-time support and feedback, enabling more personalized and responsive care. As healthcare continues to evolve, the application of AI in tailoring treatments will be fundamental in driving the future of personalized medicine, ultimately leading to better health outcomes and enhanced patient satisfaction.

Ethical Considerations in Personalized Medicine

Ethical considerations in personalized medicine are crucial as advancements in AI-driven diagnostics and treatment approaches raise various moral and ethical dilemmas. Personalized medicine holds the promise of tailoring medical treatment to individual characteristics, but this customization also brings to light issues related to patient autonomy, informed consent, and the potential for discrimination. Healthcare professionals must navigate these complexities to ensure that their practices align with ethical standards while leveraging innovative technologies.

One primary ethical concern is the need for informed consent in the context of personalized medicine. Patients often do not fully understand the implications of genetic testing and the use of AI algorithms in their treatment plans. It is essential for healthcare providers to communicate clearly about the benefits, risks, and limitations associated with personalized medicine. This includes explaining how AI-driven diagnostics work and the extent to which their data will be used. Ensuring that patients are equipped with adequate information empowers them to make informed choices about their healthcare, fostering trust in the physician-patient relationship.

Data privacy and security represent another significant ethical consideration. Personalized medicine relies heavily on vast amounts of patient data, including sensitive genetic information. The potential for data breaches or misuse raises concerns about patient confidentiality and the ethical use of such data. Healthcare organizations must implement robust data protection measures and adhere to regulations to safeguard patient information. Additionally, transparency about how data is collected, stored, and utilized is vital in maintaining public trust and ensuring compliance with ethical standards.

Equity in access to personalized medicine also warrants attention. As AI technologies advance, there is a risk that disparities in healthcare access may widen, particularly for marginalized populations. Ensuring equitable access to AI-driven diagnostic tools and personalized treatments is imperative to avoid reinforcing existing health inequalities. Policymakers and healthcare administrators must work collaboratively to create frameworks that promote inclusivity and ensure that advancements in personalized medicine benefit all segments of the population.

Finally, the potential for bias in AI algorithms poses ethical challenges that must be addressed. If the data used to train AI systems is not representative of diverse populations, the resulting algorithms may lead to inaccurate diagnoses or ineffective treatment plans for certain groups. It is essential for developers and researchers to critically evaluate the datasets used in AI development and to implement strategies that mitigate bias. Regular audits and updates of AI systems can help ensure that they remain fair and effective across different patient demographics. By addressing these ethical considerations, the healthcare community can harness the power of personalized medicine responsibly and equitably.

Chapter 4: AI in Medical Imaging Analysis

Importance of Medical Imaging

Medical imaging plays a pivotal role in modern healthcare, serving as a cornerstone for accurate diagnosis, treatment planning, and ongoing patient management. Techniques such as X-rays, CT scans, MRIs, and ultrasounds provide invaluable insights into the human body, allowing healthcare professionals to visualize internal structures and detect abnormalities that may not be apparent through physical examination alone. The precision and clarity offered by these imaging modalities facilitate early disease detection, which is crucial for conditions like cancer or cardiovascular diseases, ultimately leading to improved patient outcomes and survival rates.

The integration of artificial intelligence in medical imaging analysis is revolutionizing the field, enhancing the capabilities of traditional imaging techniques. AI algorithms can process vast amounts of imaging data with remarkable speed and accuracy, identifying patterns and anomalies that may be missed by the human eye. This technological advancement not only aids radiologists in making more informed decisions but also reduces the likelihood of diagnostic errors, thereby increasing the overall quality of care. Furthermore, AI-driven imaging tools can assist in triaging patients, prioritizing cases based on urgency and complexity, which is especially beneficial in resource-limited settings.

Personalized medicine is significantly influenced by advancements in medical imaging, as it allows for more tailored treatment approaches. By leveraging AI analysis of imaging data, healthcare providers can gain a deeper understanding of individual patient characteristics, leading to more effective and customized therapeutic strategies. For instance, in oncology, imaging assessments combined with AI can help determine the most appropriate treatment regimen for a particular tumor type, taking into account its unique biological behavior and response to therapy. This personalization not only enhances treatment efficacy but also minimizes unnecessary interventions, ultimately improving patient satisfaction and quality of life.

Moreover, the role of medical imaging extends beyond diagnosis and treatment. It is instrumental in predictive analytics, helping healthcare professionals forecast disease progression and outcomes. AI algorithms can analyze historical imaging data alongside other clinical parameters to predict future health events, enabling proactive patient management. This predictive capability is particularly valuable in chronic disease management, where timely interventions can prevent complications and reduce healthcare costs. As healthcare systems increasingly shift towards value-based care, the importance of predictive analytics in medical imaging becomes even more pronounced.

Finally, the ongoing evolution of telemedicine highlights the critical role of medical imaging in remote patient care. AI-enhanced telemedicine solutions can facilitate real-time access to imaging data, enabling healthcare providers to collaborate and consult with specialists regardless of geographic barriers. This capability not only improves healthcare accessibility but also ensures that patients receive timely interventions based on comprehensive imaging assessments. As the demand for remote healthcare continues to rise, the integration of AI in medical imaging will play a crucial role in shaping the future of patient care, fostering a more efficient and effective healthcare system.

AI Techniques in Imaging Analysis

AI techniques in imaging analysis have revolutionized the way healthcare professionals diagnose and treat patients. By leveraging advanced algorithms and machine learning models, AI can analyze medical images such as X-rays, MRIs, and CT scans with unprecedented speed and accuracy. This capability not only enhances diagnostic precision but also empowers physicians to make informed decisions quickly, ultimately improving patient outcomes. As AI continues to evolve, its integration into imaging analysis offers a glimpse into a future where diagnostic processes are more reliable and efficient.

Future Trends in Imaging Technology

Advancements in imaging technology are poised to revolutionize the landscape of healthcare, particularly through the integration of artificial intelligence. Emerging trends indicate a shift towards more sophisticated imaging modalities that leverage AI algorithms for enhanced diagnostic accuracy and efficiency. With the capacity to analyze vast datasets in real-time, AI-driven imaging systems are expected to reduce the time required for diagnoses and improve treatment outcomes. Technologies such as deep learning and computer vision are already being implemented to assist radiologists in identifying anomalies and classifying imaging data, making the process faster and more reliable.

One of the most significant trends is the development of personalized medicine through imaging. AI algorithms are increasingly capable of integrating genetic, clinical, and imaging data to create tailored treatment plans for patients. This holistic approach enables healthcare providers to understand the unique characteristics of a patient's condition, leading to more precise interventions. For instance, AI can analyze imaging studies alongside genomic data to predict how a patient will respond to specific therapies, ultimately paving the way for more effective and individualized care.

Moreover, the role of AI in medical imaging analysis is expanding beyond traditional modalities such as X-rays and MRIs. Advanced imaging techniques, including functional MRI and positron emission tomography (PET), are being enhanced through AI tools that enable the extraction of detailed insights from complex datasets. These advancements not only facilitate earlier detection of diseases but also improve monitoring of treatment responses. The integration of AI algorithms into imaging workflows is helping to create a seamless experience for clinicians, allowing them to focus on patient care while technology handles the heavy lifting of data analysis.

Predictive analytics powered by AI is another key trend that is transforming imaging technology. By analyzing historical imaging data, AI systems can identify patterns that may indicate potential health risks, enabling proactive measures. This predictive capability is particularly valuable in areas such as oncology, where early detection can significantly impact patient outcomes. Additionally, AI-driven predictive models can aid in resource allocation within healthcare facilities, optimizing workflow and enhancing operational efficiency by anticipating patient needs based on imaging trends.

Lastly, the rise of telemedicine is intertwined with advancements in imaging technology, fueled by AI enhancements. Remote diagnostics, supported by high-quality imaging and AI analysis, allow healthcare providers to consult and diagnose patients from afar. This trend not only expands access to care for underserved populations but also facilitates continuous monitoring and support for patients managing chronic conditions. AI-driven telemedicine solutions are becoming integral to mental health support, enabling providers to analyze behavioral patterns through imaging and other data sources, offering timely interventions that can improve patient well-being. As these technologies continue to evolve, they promise to significantly enhance the quality and accessibility of healthcare services across a range of specialties.

Chapter 5: AI for Predictive Analytics in Patient Care

Fundamentals of Predictive Analytics

Predictive analytics is a vital component in the evolution of healthcare, leveraging historical data and advanced algorithms to forecast future outcomes and trends. At its core, predictive analytics involves the use of statistical techniques and machine learning to analyze current and past data, allowing healthcare professionals to anticipate patient needs, improve clinical decision-making, and enhance the overall quality of care. By transforming raw data into actionable insights, predictive analytics empowers physicians and healthcare administrators to optimize resource allocation, manage patient populations more effectively, and ultimately improve patient outcomes.

One of the most significant applications of predictive analytics in healthcare is in the realm of patient care management. By analyzing patient data, including demographics, clinical history, and social determinants of health, predictive models can identify patients at high risk for conditions such as chronic diseases or hospital readmissions. This insight enables healthcare providers to implement proactive measures, such as targeted interventions and personalized treatment plans, aimed at improving patient health and reducing costs. Furthermore, predictive analytics can enhance the management of patient flow within healthcare facilities, ensuring that resources are allocated efficiently and that patients receive timely care.

In the domain of personalized medicine, predictive analytics plays a crucial role by enabling tailored treatment strategies based on individual patient profiles. Through the integration of genomic data, lifestyle factors, and past treatment responses, predictive models can guide clinicians in selecting the most effective therapies for their patients. This individualized approach not only increases the likelihood of successful outcomes but also minimizes the risk of adverse effects associated with one-size-fits-all treatments. As more data becomes available, the accuracy and efficacy of predictive models in personalizing patient care are expected to improve, paving the way for a new era in healthcare.

Predictive analytics also finds significant application in medical imaging analysis, where AI-driven tools can assist in diagnosing conditions by analyzing imaging data. By training algorithms on vast datasets of radiological images, healthcare professionals can benefit from enhanced diagnostic accuracy and speed. Predictive models can help identify subtle patterns and anomalies that may be missed by the human eye, leading to earlier detection of diseases such as cancer. As these technologies continue to advance, the integration of predictive analytics into imaging workflows is anticipated to revolutionize how radiologists interpret images and inform treatment decisions.

Finally, the integration of predictive analytics into AI-enhanced telemedicine solutions exemplifies its transformative potential in healthcare delivery. By leveraging patient data collected through remote monitoring devices and telehealth platforms, predictive models can facilitate timely interventions and support ongoing patient engagement. This is particularly beneficial in managing chronic conditions, where continuous monitoring and real-time feedback can significantly improve patient adherence to treatment plans. As telemedicine continues to expand, the role of predictive analytics in ensuring effective remote care will be essential in supporting patient health and optimizing healthcare resources.

AI Models in Patient Outcome Prediction

AI models have become pivotal in transforming patient outcome prediction, offering healthcare professionals tools to better understand and anticipate patient needs. By leveraging large datasets, these models can analyze complex patterns in patient data, including historical health records, demographic information, and clinical indicators. This predictive capability allows for improved decision-making processes, enabling healthcare providers to identify at-risk patients earlier and intervene proactively. As a result, AI-driven predictions facilitate personalized treatment plans that cater specifically to individual patient profiles.

Various AI techniques, including machine learning and deep learning, are employed to refine patient outcome predictions. Machine learning algorithms can identify correlations within vast datasets, while deep learning networks are adept at processing unstructured data such as medical images and textual notes from electronic health records. These advanced methodologies can significantly enhance diagnostic accuracy and clinical forecasting, allowing for more effective allocation of resources and interventions tailored to patient needs. Continuous advancements in these technologies further enhance their applicability in real-world clinical settings.

Moreover, the integration of AI models in predictive analytics is a game changer for chronic disease management. For conditions such as diabetes and cardiovascular diseases, AI algorithms can analyze patient behaviors, treatment responses, and lifestyle factors to predict potential complications. This predictive insight empowers healthcare teams to implement preventative measures, adjust treatment protocols, and engage patients in their own care, leading to better health outcomes and reduced hospital readmissions. The shift towards data-driven approaches signifies a move away from reactive care models to a more proactive and personalized healthcare paradigm.

In addition to improving patient outcomes, AI models in predictive analytics contribute to operational efficiencies within healthcare systems. By predicting patient flow and resource utilization, healthcare administrators can optimize staffing levels and reduce waiting times, enhancing the overall patient experience. Furthermore, predictive modeling can assist in managing healthcare costs by pinpointing areas where interventions can prevent more expensive treatments down the line. This dual benefit of enhanced patient care and operational optimization makes AI models an essential asset in modern healthcare management.

Finally, the ethical implications and challenges surrounding AI in patient outcome prediction must be addressed. As AI systems become more integrated into clinical workflows, concerns regarding data privacy, algorithmic bias, and transparency arise. It is imperative for healthcare professionals and data scientists to collaborate, ensuring that AI implementations are not only effective but also equitable and responsible. Through rigorous validation and adherence to ethical guidelines, the healthcare sector can harness the full potential of AI models to improve patient outcomes while safeguarding patient trust and privacy.

Enhancing Patient Management with AI

The integration of artificial intelligence (AI) into healthcare practices has the potential to revolutionize patient management, streamlining processes and improving outcomes. AI-driven diagnostic tools can analyze vast amounts of patient data, enabling healthcare providers to make more accurate and timely decisions. By leveraging machine learning algorithms, these tools can identify patterns and anomalies in medical imaging, lab results, and patient history that may not be readily apparent to human observers. This capability enhances diagnostic accuracy and reduces the time required to arrive at critical decisions, ultimately leading to better patient care.

Personalized medicine is another domain where AI plays a crucial role. By harnessing data from electronic health records, genetic information, and lifestyle factors, AI can help tailor treatment plans to individual patients. This personalized approach enhances the efficacy of interventions, as therapies can be optimized based on the specific characteristics and needs of each patient. Furthermore, predictive analytics powered by AI can anticipate potential health issues before they arise, allowing for proactive measures that can prevent complications and improve long-term health outcomes.

AI-enhanced telemedicine solutions are transforming how healthcare providers engage with patients, especially in remote or underserved areas. Through AI-driven platforms, physicians can conduct virtual consultations, monitor patient compliance, and manage chronic conditions more effectively. These solutions not only improve access to care but also facilitate continuous patient engagement, providing real-time feedback and support. As AI technologies evolve, they will continue to enhance telemedicine, making it a staple in modern healthcare delivery.

In the realm of mental health, AI is proving invaluable for monitoring and support. AI algorithms can analyze patient interactions, assess mood changes, and identify risk factors associated with mental health issues. By processing data from various sources, including wearable devices and social media activity, AI can provide insights that inform care strategies. This approach enables mental health professionals to offer timely interventions and support tailored to individual patients, fostering a more responsive and effective care environment.

As AI continues to advance, its applications in drug discovery and development are becoming increasingly relevant. By utilizing AI to analyze biological data, researchers can identify potential therapeutic targets and predict the efficacy of new compounds. This accelerates the drug development process, reducing the time and cost associated with bringing new medications to market. The synergy between AI and healthcare not only enhances patient management but also fosters innovation that can lead to groundbreaking treatments and improved health outcomes across the spectrum of care.

Chapter 6: AI-Based Drug Discovery and Development

Overview of Drug Discovery Process

The drug discovery process is a complex and multifaceted journey that typically spans several stages, integrating various scientific disciplines and technologies. At its core, the process begins with the identification of potential drug targets, often proteins or genes implicated in disease pathways. Researchers employ high-throughput screening techniques to evaluate vast libraries of compounds for their ability to interact with these targets. This initial phase is crucial, as it sets the foundation for subsequent development stages. Advances in computational biology and bioinformatics have significantly enhanced our ability to predict which compounds may be most effective, thereby streamlining the selection process.

Once promising compounds are identified, they undergo a rigorous optimization phase. Medicinal chemistry plays a pivotal role here, where chemists modify the chemical structure of lead compounds to improve their efficacy, reduce toxicity, and enhance pharmacokinetic properties. This iterative process often involves synthesizing numerous analogs and testing them in vitro and in vivo. The integration of AI-driven approaches, such as machine learning algorithms, can accelerate this phase by predicting the outcomes of chemical modifications and identifying optimal candidates for further development.

Following optimization, the selected drug candidates progress to preclinical and clinical trials. Preclinical studies assess the safety and biological activity of the compounds in animal models, while clinical trials encompass three phases of human testing to evaluate safety, dosage, and efficacy. The use of AI tools in this stage can provide predictive analytics to identify patient populations that may benefit most from the treatment and optimize trial designs. AI can also enhance patient monitoring through advanced imaging techniques and electronic health records, ensuring that data is collected efficiently and analyzed for potential insights.

Regulatory approval is the next critical step in the drug discovery process. The submission of comprehensive data to regulatory bodies, such as the FDA, involves demonstrating that the drug is safe and effective for its intended use. AI technologies can assist in this phase by automating data analysis, improving the accuracy of submissions, and ensuring compliance with regulatory standards. Moreover, AI can facilitate post-market surveillance, allowing for ongoing monitoring of drug safety and efficacy in the general population.

Finally, the entire drug discovery process is increasingly influenced by personalized medicine approaches, where patient-specific factors guide therapeutic decisions. AI-driven diagnostic tools enable healthcare providers to tailor treatments based on genetic, environmental, and lifestyle factors unique to each patient. This shift towards personalized medicine not only improves patient outcomes but also enhances the efficiency of drug development by focusing resources on the most promising therapeutic avenues. As the field continues to evolve, the integration of AI technologies will likely redefine traditional drug discovery paradigms, leading to faster, safer, and more effective therapeutic options.

AI's Role in Accelerating Drug Development

AI's integration into drug development has revolutionized the pharmaceutical landscape, streamlining processes that traditionally spanned years or even decades. By leveraging machine learning algorithms and vast datasets, AI can predict how different compounds will interact with biological systems, significantly reducing the time required for initial screening and validation. This capability not only accelerates the identification of promising drug candidates but also minimizes the reliance on costly and time-consuming laboratory experiments, allowing researchers to focus resources on the most viable options.

Moreover, AI-driven analytics facilitate a deeper understanding of disease mechanisms, enabling the design of more targeted therapies. By analyzing genetic information and patient data, AI can identify biomarkers and predict patient responses to specific treatments. This personalized approach not only enhances the efficacy of drugs but also improves patient safety by reducing adverse reactions associated with ineffective treatments. As healthcare moves toward a model centered on individualized care, AI's role in tailoring drug development to patient profiles becomes increasingly vital.

In the realm of clinical trials, AI enhances efficiency by optimizing trial designs and participant selection. Traditional trials often face challenges related to recruitment and retention, leading to delays and increased costs. AI can analyze vast amounts of patient data to identify suitable candidates based on specific eligibility criteria, ensuring that trials are populated with the right participants. Additionally, AI tools can monitor trial progress in real-time, providing insights that help adapt protocols and address issues as they arise, thereby enhancing the likelihood of successful outcomes.

AI also plays a crucial role in post-market surveillance, where it monitors the safety and effectiveness of drugs once they are available to the public. By analyzing data from electronic health records, social media, and other sources, AI can detect patterns that may indicate adverse effects or long-term complications associated with a drug. This continuous monitoring not only protects patients but also informs regulatory bodies and pharmaceutical companies about necessary modifications or withdrawals of medications, ensuring a higher standard of care.

As AI technology continues to evolve, its applications in drug development will expand even further. Innovations in natural language processing and deep learning are paving the way for more sophisticated analyses of scientific literature and clinical data, potentially uncovering new therapeutic targets and drug repurposing opportunities. For healthcare professionals, understanding and embracing these advancements will be essential in harnessing AI's full potential, ultimately transforming drug development into a more efficient, effective, and patient-centered process.

Successful AI Applications in Drug Discovery

Successful AI applications in drug discovery have marked a significant turning point in the pharmaceutical landscape, demonstrating the potential of artificial intelligence to streamline and enhance the drug development process. Traditional drug discovery is often lengthy and fraught with high failure rates, but AI-driven methodologies have introduced innovative approaches that can analyze vast datasets, identify patterns, and predict outcomes more accurately than ever before. These advancements have not only reduced the time required to bring new therapies to market but also improved the likelihood of their success, ultimately benefiting patients and healthcare providers alike.

One of the most promising uses of AI in drug discovery is in the identification of potential drug candidates through computational methods. Machine learning algorithms can analyze chemical databases and biological data to uncover novel compounds that may interact with specific targets in the body. This approach allows researchers to rapidly screen thousands of potential drugs in silico, significantly decreasing the need for time-consuming laboratory experiments. By leveraging AI, pharmaceutical companies can focus their resources on the most promising candidates, improving efficiency and lowering costs in the early stages of drug development.

Moreover, AI applications extend beyond candidate identification; they also play a crucial role in optimizing drug formulations and predicting their pharmacokinetics and toxicity profiles. AI-driven models can simulate how drugs behave in the human body, providing insights into absorption, distribution, metabolism, and excretion. This predictive capability is vital for ensuring drug safety and efficacy, as it allows researchers to identify adverse effects before clinical trials begin. As a result, AI not only accelerates the discovery process but also enhances the quality of new medications, ultimately safeguarding patient health.

Collaborative efforts between AI developers and pharmaceutical researchers have yielded significant breakthroughs in personalized medicine. By integrating genomic data, patient health records, and real-world evidence, AI can help identify biomarkers that predict how different patients will respond to specific treatments. This personalized approach to drug discovery ensures that therapies are tailored to individual patient profiles, improving treatment outcomes and minimizing adverse effects. Such advancements are crucial in managing complex diseases, where a one-size-fits-all approach is often ineffective.

The ongoing evolution of AI in drug discovery continues to promise transformative changes for the healthcare industry. As AI technologies become more sophisticated, their applications in drug development are expected to expand further, leading to the discovery of innovative therapies for previously untreatable conditions. As doctors, researchers, and healthcare administrators embrace these tools, the potential for improved patient care through AI-driven drug discovery will become increasingly evident, paving the way for a new era of personalized and effective medicine.

Chapter 7: AI-Enhanced Telemedicine Solutions

Telemedicine Landscape

The telemedicine landscape has undergone significant transformation in recent years, driven largely by advancements in technology and an increasing demand for accessible healthcare. The integration of artificial intelligence into telemedicine frameworks has enhanced the delivery of care, enabling healthcare providers to reach patients in remote areas and reduce barriers to access. This shift not only improves healthcare outcomes but also streamlines the diagnostic process, allowing for quicker decision-making and treatment initiation. As a result, telemedicine has become a vital component of modern healthcare systems, particularly in the wake of global health crises that have highlighted the need for innovative solutions.

AI-driven diagnostic tools are at the forefront of this evolution, providing clinicians with advanced capabilities to analyze patient data efficiently. These tools assist in identifying patterns and anomalies in patient health records, leading to more accurate diagnoses. For instance, AI algorithms can process extensive datasets derived from telemedicine consultations, enabling physicians to pinpoint potential health issues that may not be immediately apparent through traditional assessment methods. The synergy between telemedicine and AI fosters a proactive approach to patient care, where early detection and intervention can significantly improve health outcomes.

Personalized medicine is another area significantly impacted by the advancements in telemedicine and AI. By leveraging data analytics and machine learning algorithms, healthcare providers can tailor treatment plans based on individual patient profiles, including genetic information, lifestyle factors, and medical history. This level of customization ensures that patients receive the most effective therapies while minimizing potential side effects. The ability to deliver personalized care remotely not only enhances patient satisfaction but also promotes adherence to treatment regimens, as patients feel more engaged and invested in their health journey.

AI's role in medical imaging analysis has also expanded within the telemedicine landscape, allowing for remote interpretation of diagnostic images. With the aid of AI algorithms, healthcare professionals can analyze radiographs, MRIs, and CT scans more accurately and swiftly, facilitating timely interventions. This capability is particularly beneficial in rural or underserved areas where access to specialized radiologists may be limited. The integration of AI in telemedicine not only enhances the quality of diagnostic imaging but also ensures that patients receive critical care without unnecessary delays, ultimately saving lives.

As the telemedicine landscape continues to evolve, the potential for AI-enhanced solutions to address mental health monitoring and support is becoming increasingly apparent. Teletherapy platforms utilizing AI can analyze patient interactions and provide real-time insights to clinicians, helping them assess emotional states and tailor therapeutic approaches. These platforms also offer patients greater flexibility in accessing mental health resources, which is essential in a world where mental health issues are on the rise. By harnessing the power of AI in telemedicine, healthcare providers can create a more holistic and responsive approach to patient care, ensuring that all aspects of health—physical and mental—are addressed in a comprehensive manner.

AI Tools for Remote Patient Monitoring

The integration of artificial intelligence in remote patient monitoring (RPM) represents a significant advancement in the healthcare industry, facilitating continuous patient observation outside traditional clinical settings. These AI tools enhance the ability to collect, analyze, and interpret vast amounts of health data in real time, thereby improving patient outcomes and allowing healthcare providers to deliver personalized care. By utilizing various sensors, wearables, and mobile applications, AI systems can track vital signs, detect anomalies, and alert healthcare professionals to potential issues, ensuring timely interventions.

One of the prominent features of AI-powered RPM systems is their ability to leverage machine learning algorithms to analyze patient data. These algorithms can identify patterns and trends that may not be immediately apparent to human observers. For instance, they can track changes in a patient's heart rate, blood pressure, or glucose levels over time, providing insights that help in managing chronic conditions. By using predictive analytics, these tools can effectively forecast potential health crises, allowing physicians to intervene before a patient's condition deteriorates significantly.

AI tools also play a crucial role in enhancing patient engagement and adherence to treatment plans. Many RPM platforms incorporate personalized messaging and reminders, which help patients stay on track with their medications and lifestyle changes. These systems often use natural language processing to facilitate communication, allowing patients to interact with the technology in a more intuitive manner. By fostering a collaborative relationship between patients and healthcare providers, AI tools can improve compliance rates and empower patients to take an active role in their health management.

In addition to improving individual patient care, AI-driven RPM tools are invaluable for aggregating data at a population level. This capability enables healthcare administrators and researchers to analyze health trends across diverse groups, leading to improved public health strategies and resource allocation. By harnessing big data analytics, these tools can help identify at-risk populations, evaluate the effectiveness of interventions, and guide future research directions. Consequently, the insights gained from these analyses can support evidence-based decision-making in healthcare policies and practices.

As the adoption of AI in remote patient monitoring continues to grow, it presents unique opportunities for interdisciplinary collaboration among healthcare professionals, engineers, and data scientists. The successful implementation of these technologies relies on a shared understanding of clinical needs and technical capabilities. By bringing together expertise from various fields, stakeholders can develop innovative solutions that address the complexities of patient monitoring, ultimately leading to a more efficient and responsive healthcare system. The future of RPM lies in the synergy between AI technologies and the clinical insights of healthcare providers, paving the way for a more proactive and patient-centered approach to medical care.

Improving Patient Engagement Through AI

Improving patient engagement through artificial intelligence (AI) represents a significant advancement in healthcare, enhancing both the quality of care and the patient experience. AI-driven tools are increasingly being utilized to create personalized interactions with patients, allowing for tailored communication and support. With the integration of AI systems, healthcare providers can better understand individual patient needs, preferences, and behaviors. This data-driven approach not only fosters a stronger doctor-patient relationship but also empowers patients to take an active role in their own health management.

AI technologies facilitate the collection and analysis of vast amounts of patient data, which can be used to identify trends and patterns that inform treatment plans. For instance, predictive analytics can forecast potential health issues based on a patient's medical history and lifestyle choices, enabling proactive interventions. By leveraging AI in this manner, healthcare professionals can engage patients more effectively, guiding them through treatment options and encouraging adherence to prescribed therapies. This increased engagement can lead to improved health outcomes and a reduction in hospital readmissions.

In the realm of telemedicine, AI-driven platforms are revolutionizing patient engagement by providing remote access to healthcare services. Through virtual consultations powered by AI, patients can receive timely medical advice without the barriers of distance or mobility. These platforms often incorporate chatbots and virtual assistants that can answer patient queries, schedule appointments, and offer health tips based on individual conditions. This immediate access to information and support enhances patient satisfaction and encourages regular interaction with healthcare providers, ultimately leading to better health management.

AI's role in mental health monitoring and support is another critical area for improving patient engagement. Machine learning algorithms can analyze data from wearables and mobile applications to track patients' emotional and psychological well-being. By identifying patterns in behavior or mood fluctuations, AI can alert healthcare providers to changes that may require intervention. This real-time monitoring not only fosters a more responsive approach to mental health care but also helps patients feel more connected and supported throughout their treatment journey.

Furthermore, as AI technologies continue to evolve, they hold the potential to democratize access to healthcare information. Educational AI tools can provide patients with personalized resources, helping them understand their conditions and treatment options in a way that is accessible and comprehensible. By equipping patients with knowledge, AI fosters a sense of autonomy, allowing them to engage more fully in their healthcare decisions. As a result, the healthcare system can shift from a reactive model to a more collaborative one, where patient engagement is at the forefront of care delivery.

Chapter 8: AI for Mental Health Monitoring and Support

Mental Health Challenges in Healthcare

Mental health challenges in healthcare significantly impact both providers and patients, often exacerbating existing issues within the medical system. Healthcare professionals frequently face high levels of stress, burnout, and mental health disorders such as anxiety and depression. The demanding nature of healthcare work, particularly in high-stakes environments like emergency rooms and intensive care units, can lead to emotional exhaustion and a diminished sense of personal accomplishment. This not only affects the well-being of healthcare workers but also compromises the quality of care they provide to patients.

The implications of these mental health challenges extend beyond individual practitioners. When healthcare workers experience burnout, it can lead to increased rates of absenteeism, decreased job satisfaction, and a heightened likelihood of making medical errors. These outcomes ultimately affect patient safety and care quality, resulting in poorer health outcomes for patients. Furthermore, the stigma surrounding mental health issues in the medical community often prevents healthcare providers from seeking the help they need, perpetuating a cycle of distress that can impact entire healthcare teams and organizations.

Incorporating AI-driven solutions can help address these challenges by providing tools for early detection and intervention for mental health issues among healthcare personnel. For instance, AI can analyze patterns in behavioral data, identifying signs of stress or burnout before they escalate into more severe conditions. These insights can empower healthcare administrators to implement preventive measures, such as wellness programs or mental health support initiatives tailored to the unique needs of their staff. By fostering a supportive work environment, healthcare organizations can mitigate the impact of mental health challenges on their workforce.

Moreover, AI can enhance the overall patient experience by providing support for mental health monitoring and intervention. With AI-powered tools, healthcare providers can track patients' mental health through continuous monitoring of relevant indicators, such as mood, sleep patterns, and social interactions. This capability enables personalized treatment plans that can adapt to the patient's evolving needs, ultimately leading to better patient engagement and outcomes. In addition, AI-driven telemedicine solutions can offer patients convenient access to mental health services, breaking down barriers related to stigma and accessibility.

As the healthcare landscape continues to evolve, addressing mental health challenges is essential for creating a sustainable, effective system. By leveraging AI technologies, healthcare stakeholders can improve the well-being of both providers and patients, cultivating a healthier, more resilient healthcare environment. Emphasizing mental health as a critical component of overall healthcare strategy not only benefits individuals but also enhances the collective capacity of the healthcare system to meet the growing demands of patient care.

AI Applications in Mental Health

AI applications in mental health are revolutionizing the way healthcare professionals diagnose, treat, and monitor patients. These advancements are particularly significant given the rising prevalence of mental health disorders globally. Traditional methods of assessment and therapy often rely on subjective evaluations and limited data, which can lead to variability in diagnosis and treatment efficacy. AI-driven tools, however, can analyze vast amounts of data from various sources, including electronic health records, social media activity, and wearable devices, to provide a more comprehensive understanding of a patient's mental health status.

One of the most promising applications of AI in mental health is the development of predictive analytics tools. These tools leverage machine learning algorithms to identify patterns and trends in patient data, enabling healthcare providers to anticipate mental health crises before they occur. By analyzing factors such as historical data, demographic information, and even real-time behavioral cues, these systems can alert clinicians to potential risks, allowing for timely interventions. This proactive approach not only enhances patient outcomes but also optimizes resource allocation within healthcare settings.

Natural language processing (NLP) is another area where AI is making significant strides in mental health care. NLP algorithms can analyze unstructured data, such as patient notes and therapy transcripts, to derive insights about patient sentiments, mood fluctuations, and treatment responses. This capability allows mental health professionals to gain deeper insights into a patient's mental state and tailor interventions accordingly. Furthermore, AI-driven chatbots and virtual therapists are being developed to provide immediate support for patients, particularly in situations where access to traditional therapy may be limited.

AI is also enhancing telemedicine solutions, which have gained prominence in mental health care, especially in the wake of the COVID-19 pandemic. These platforms utilize AI to improve the user experience, facilitate remote assessments, and provide personalized treatment recommendations based on patient interactions. For instance, AI algorithms can analyze video consultations to detect signs of distress or disengagement, prompting clinicians to adjust their approach in real-time. This integration of AI into telemedicine not only expands access to mental health services but also ensures that care is responsive to individual needs.

Lastly, AI's role in mental health extends to research and drug development. AI-based tools are being employed to identify potential therapeutic targets and predict patient responses to various treatments. By analyzing genetic, biochemical, and behavioral data, researchers can develop more effective personalized treatment plans. The ability to simulate and analyze vast datasets accelerates the pace of discovery in mental health therapeutics, ultimately leading to more innovative and effective solutions for patients suffering from mental health disorders. As these technologies continue to evolve, their integration into clinical practice holds the potential to transform mental health care delivery significantly.

Future of AI in Mental Health Services

The future of artificial intelligence in mental health services promises to revolutionize the way healthcare providers approach diagnosis, treatment, and ongoing support for patients. With the increasing prevalence of mental health issues globally, the integration of AI-driven tools into mental health services is not just beneficial but essential. These technologies can assist practitioners in identifying patterns and predicting patient outcomes more accurately than traditional methods. By leveraging vast amounts of data from diverse sources, AI can provide insights that enhance the understanding of mental health conditions, leading to more effective interventions.

AI algorithms are being developed to analyze speech patterns, facial expressions, and even physiological responses to assess mental health status. Such tools can serve as early warning systems for conditions like depression and anxiety, allowing healthcare providers to intervene before symptoms escalate. Machine learning models trained on extensive datasets can recognize subtle changes in behavior that may indicate a decline in mental health, enabling timely and personalized care. Moreover, these algorithms can continually learn from new data, refining their predictive capabilities and ultimately improving patient outcomes.

Telemedicine, enhanced by AI, is set to play a pivotal role in mental health services. Virtual consultations powered by AI algorithms can facilitate real-time assessments and recommendations, making mental health care more accessible to those in remote or underserved areas. AI-driven chatbots and virtual assistants can provide immediate support, offering coping strategies and resources outside of traditional therapy hours. This technology not only expands access to care but also reduces the stigma associated with seeking mental health treatment, encouraging more individuals to engage with available services.

Personalized medicine, a key focus of AI in healthcare, is particularly relevant to mental health. By analyzing genetic, environmental, and lifestyle factors, AI can help tailor treatment plans to individual patients. This approach ensures that interventions are more aligned with the unique characteristics of each patient, potentially leading to more effective outcomes. Furthermore, AI can facilitate the discovery of new therapeutic approaches by identifying previously unrecognized relationships between various factors and mental health conditions, paving the way for innovative treatment options.

As we look to the future, the ethical considerations surrounding the use of AI in mental health services must be addressed. Ensuring patient privacy, maintaining data security, and avoiding algorithmic bias are crucial for building trust in these technologies. Collaborative efforts among healthcare providers, researchers, and technology developers will be essential to create robust frameworks that guide the responsible use of AI in mental health. Ultimately, the integration of AI into mental health services holds the potential to enhance the quality of care, improve patient outcomes, and foster a more holistic approach to mental wellness in the healthcare landscape.

Chapter 9: Challenges and Limitations of AI in Healthcare

Data Privacy and Security Concerns

Data privacy and security concerns are paramount in the integration of artificial intelligence within healthcare systems. As AI-driven diagnostics become more prevalent, the volume of sensitive patient data being processed and analyzed increases significantly. This data often includes personal health information, medical histories, and genetic information, all of which are protected under various regulations such as HIPAA in the United States. Failure to adequately secure this data can lead to serious implications, including breaches of patient confidentiality, legal repercussions for healthcare providers, and loss of trust in AI technologies among patients and practitioners alike.

The potential for data breaches is exacerbated by the interconnected nature of modern healthcare systems. As healthcare providers adopt AI technologies, the need for interoperability between different systems becomes critical. However, this interconnectedness can create vulnerabilities, making it easier for cybercriminals to exploit weaknesses in security protocols. Consequently, healthcare organizations must implement robust cybersecurity measures, including encryption, access controls, and regular security audits, to protect patient data from unauthorized access and cyber-attacks.

Moreover, the ethical implications surrounding data privacy in AI applications cannot be overlooked. The use of AI in personalized medicine, for instance, necessitates the collection and analysis of extensive datasets that may include identifiable patient information. Researchers and developers must balance the benefits of AI-driven insights with the ethical responsibility to protect individual privacy. This includes ensuring that data is anonymized when possible and obtaining informed consent from patients before their data is used for research or diagnostic purposes. The establishment of clear ethical guidelines and frameworks is essential to navigate these challenges.

In addition to ethical considerations, the rapid advancement of AI technologies can outpace existing regulatory frameworks. Policymakers and regulatory bodies are often struggling to keep up with the innovations that AI brings to the healthcare sector, which can lead to gray areas in compliance and governance. Healthcare organizations must actively engage with regulators to shape policies that adequately address data privacy and security concerns while fostering innovation. Collaborative efforts between stakeholders, including healthcare providers, technology companies, and regulatory agencies, are crucial to establishing standards that protect patient data without stifling progress.

Finally, continuous education and training for healthcare professionals on data privacy and security practices are vital. As AI technologies evolve, so do the methods employed by malicious actors seeking to exploit vulnerabilities. By cultivating a culture of awareness and vigilance among doctors, nurses, and administrators, healthcare organizations can enhance their defenses against security threats. Incorporating data privacy training into medical and engineering curricula will also prepare the next generation of professionals to prioritize security in their work with AI-driven tools, ultimately ensuring that patient care remains safe and effective in an increasingly digital landscape.

Integration with Existing Systems

Integration with existing systems in healthcare is a critical consideration for the successful implementation of AI-driven diagnostics. The healthcare landscape is characterized by a multitude of legacy systems, electronic health records (EHR), and various diagnostic tools that have been developed over the years. The challenge lies in ensuring that new AI technologies can seamlessly interface with these existing infrastructures. A well-planned integration strategy not only enhances the functionality of AI tools but also ensures that healthcare professionals can utilize them without disrupting their workflow. The alignment of AI systems with established practices is essential for fostering acceptance among clinicians and improving patient outcomes.

One of the primary objectives of integrating AI-driven diagnostics is to streamline data flow across disparate systems. Healthcare providers often work with various software platforms that handle everything from patient registration to lab results and imaging. AI applications can enhance these processes by providing real-time analytics and insights derived from comprehensive patient data. For example, an AI diagnostic tool can analyze imaging results and suggest potential diagnoses, all while pulling relevant patient history from EHR systems. This capability not only improves the efficiency of care delivery but also enhances the accuracy of diagnoses, thus reducing the likelihood of human error.

Moreover, the integration of AI with existing systems facilitates personalized medicine. By leveraging vast amounts of patient data, AI algorithms can identify patterns and correlations that are not readily apparent to clinicians. This integration allows for the development of tailored treatment plans based on individual patient profiles, including genetic information and lifestyle factors. For healthcare providers, the ability to access integrated AI insights directly within their existing systems empowers them to make more informed decisions, thereby improving the quality of care. Ultimately, personalized medicine through AI can lead to better health outcomes and a more patient-centered approach.

Another crucial aspect of integrating AI-driven diagnostics is ensuring compliance with healthcare regulations and standards. As organizations adopt AI technologies, they must navigate a complex landscape of legal and ethical considerations, including data privacy, security, and patient consent. Integrating AI solutions with existing systems requires a thorough understanding of these regulations to ensure that patient data is handled responsibly. Healthcare administrators must work closely with IT professionals to implement robust security measures and establish protocols for data usage that comply with regulations such as HIPAA. This compliance not only protects patient information but also builds trust among patients and healthcare providers.

Lastly, the integration process is not solely a technical challenge; it also involves cultural and organizational change within healthcare institutions. For successful adoption, healthcare professionals must be trained on how to leverage AI tools within their existing workflows effectively. This requires a commitment to continuous education and a willingness to adapt to new technologies. By fostering a culture of innovation and collaboration, healthcare organizations can create an environment where AI-driven diagnostics are viewed as valuable assets rather than burdens. Engaging all stakeholders in the integration process, including doctors, nurses, and administrative staff, can enhance the overall acceptance and utilization of AI technologies in healthcare.

Addressing Bias in AI Algorithms

Addressing bias in AI algorithms is crucial for ensuring equitable and effective healthcare outcomes. AI-driven diagnostic tools and applications are increasingly relied upon in clinical settings, where the stakes are high, and patient trust is paramount. However, if these systems are trained on biased data, they can perpetuate existing disparities in healthcare. Bias can manifest in various ways, including demographic imbalances in training datasets, which may lead to AI models that perform poorly for underrepresented groups. It is essential for healthcare professionals and technologists to understand these biases, recognize their potential consequences, and actively work to mitigate them.

To effectively address bias, it is vital to ensure that AI systems are developed using comprehensive datasets that accurately reflect the diversity of the patient population. This includes considering factors such as race, gender, age, and socioeconomic status. By incorporating diverse data sources, researchers and developers can create algorithms that are more representative and capable of accurately diagnosing and treating a wide range of patients. Furthermore, continuous monitoring and evaluation of AI algorithms in real-world settings can help identify performance discrepancies among different demographic groups, allowing for timely adjustments to improve equity in patient care.

Transparency in AI algorithms is another critical component of addressing bias. Healthcare professionals must be able to understand how AI systems arrive at their conclusions to ensure that they can trust and effectively utilize these tools in practice. This can be achieved through explainable AI techniques, which provide insights into the decision-making processes of algorithms. By fostering an environment where transparency is prioritized, healthcare providers can be more confident in the recommendations made by AI systems, leading to better clinical decisions and improved patient outcomes.

Collaboration between healthcare professionals and data scientists is essential in mitigating bias within AI algorithms. By fostering interdisciplinary partnerships, stakeholders can share their unique perspectives and expertise, leading to the development of more robust and unbiased AI solutions. For instance, physicians can provide valuable insights into clinical workflows and the nuances of patient care, while data scientists can offer technical knowledge on algorithm design and data management. This collaborative approach not only enhances the quality of AI-driven diagnostic tools but also promotes a more holistic understanding of patient needs.

Finally, education and awareness play critical roles in combating bias in AI algorithms. Training programs for medical professionals, computer scientists, and engineers should incorporate discussions on the ethical implications of AI in healthcare, emphasizing the importance of fairness and accountability. By cultivating a culture of vigilance against bias, the healthcare community can ensure that AI technologies are developed and implemented in ways that promote health equity and improve patient care. As AI continues to evolve, it is imperative that all stakeholders remain committed to addressing bias proactively, creating a future where AI serves as a tool for enhancing healthcare for all individuals.

Chapter 10: The Future of AI in Healthcare

Emerging Trends and Technologies

The landscape of healthcare is rapidly evolving, driven by the advent of artificial intelligence (AI) and its myriad applications in diagnostics and patient care. Emerging trends reveal a significant shift towards AI-driven diagnostic tools that enhance accuracy and efficiency in clinical settings. These tools leverage machine learning algorithms to analyze vast datasets, enabling physicians to make informed decisions based on real-time data. The integration of AI into diagnostic processes not only streamlines workflows but also reduces human error, ultimately leading to improved patient outcomes.

One notable trend is the rise of personalized medicine, which tailors treatment plans to individual patient profiles. AI facilitates this approach by analyzing genetic, environmental, and lifestyle data to determine the most effective therapies for specific patient populations. This shift towards precision medicine signifies a departure from the traditional one-size-fits-all model, allowing healthcare providers to optimize treatment efficacy and minimize adverse effects. As AI technologies continue to mature, the ability to deliver personalized care will become increasingly sophisticated, enhancing patient engagement and satisfaction.

In the realm of medical imaging analysis, AI is transforming the way practitioners interpret complex imaging data. Advanced algorithms can detect anomalies that may be overlooked by the human eye, thereby improving early diagnosis of conditions such as cancer and cardiovascular diseases. The integration of AI in imaging not only accelerates the diagnostic process but also supports radiologists in making more accurate assessments. As these technologies advance, the potential for AI to assist in real-time imaging interpretation will further enhance clinical decision-making capabilities.

Predictive analytics powered by AI is another emerging trend that holds promise for proactive patient care. By analyzing historical patient data, AI models can identify patterns and predict potential health risks, allowing healthcare providers to intervene before conditions escalate. This proactive approach not only improves patient outcomes but also optimizes resource allocation within healthcare systems. As predictive modeling becomes more refined, its integration into routine clinical practice will empower physicians to deliver timely and targeted interventions.

Finally, AI-enhanced telemedicine solutions are on the rise, enabling remote patient monitoring and support. These tools facilitate continuous communication between patients and healthcare providers, particularly for those with chronic conditions. AI algorithms can analyze patient-reported data to identify trends and trigger alerts for necessary follow-ups. The integration of AI in telemedicine not only expands access to care but also fosters a more personalized healthcare experience. As these technologies develop, they promise to reshape the future of healthcare delivery, ensuring that patients receive timely and effective care regardless of their location.

The Role of Healthcare Professionals in AI Development

The integration of artificial intelligence into healthcare is not solely a technological endeavor; it necessitates the active participation of healthcare professionals at every stage of development. Physicians, nurses, and medical researchers bring invaluable clinical insights that inform the design and functionality of AI-driven diagnostic tools. Their firsthand experiences with patient care, treatment protocols, and the complexities of medical conditions ensure that AI systems are not only clinically relevant but also user-friendly and aligned with the realities of healthcare practice. This collaboration helps in creating algorithms that accurately reflect the nuances of patient interactions and the variability of clinical presentations.

Healthcare professionals also play a critical role in validating AI tools. The effectiveness of AI-driven diagnostics and predictive analytics hinges on rigorous testing in real-world clinical settings. Doctors and researchers are essential in conducting studies that assess the performance of AI applications, ensuring that they meet the stringent standards required for clinical use. Their involvement extends to defining key performance indicators and evaluating outcomes, which ultimately contributes to the credibility and acceptance of AI technologies within the medical community. This validation process is crucial for gaining trust among practitioners who must rely on these tools in their day-to-day decision-making.

In the realm of personalized medicine, healthcare professionals are pivotal in guiding the development of AI systems that take into account individual patient characteristics. By providing insights into patient demographics, genetic backgrounds, and treatment responses, medical professionals help in shaping AI algorithms that can tailor interventions to specific patient needs. This collaborative approach not only enhances the accuracy of AI-driven predictions but also fosters a more patient-centered model of care. As AI continues to evolve, ongoing input from healthcare teams will be essential to refine these systems and ensure they are adaptable to diverse patient populations.

Moreover, the input of healthcare professionals is vital for the ethical implementation of AI technologies. Issues such as data privacy, informed consent, and the potential for algorithmic bias are concerns that require the expertise of medical practitioners and researchers. By participating in discussions around the ethical implications of AI, they can advocate for practices that protect patient rights while promoting innovation. Their unique perspective is crucial in establishing guidelines that govern the responsible use of AI in healthcare, ensuring that advancements are made without compromising the integrity of patient care.

Finally, as AI-driven telemedicine solutions and mental health monitoring tools gain traction, the role of healthcare professionals becomes increasingly significant. Their engagement in the design and deployment of these technologies ensures that they meet the practical needs of patients and providers alike. By providing feedback on user experience and clinical workflows, healthcare professionals can help refine these tools to enhance accessibility and effectiveness. As the landscape of healthcare continues to shift towards more technology-driven solutions, the collaboration between AI developers and healthcare practitioners will be essential in realizing the full potential of AI in transforming patient care.

Preparing for the Future: Education and Training Needs

As the landscape of healthcare continues to evolve with the integration of artificial intelligence, it becomes increasingly essential for professionals in the medical field to prepare for the future through targeted education and training. The rapid advancement of AI-driven diagnostic tools and personalized medicine necessitates a comprehensive understanding of both the technology and its applications in healthcare. This preparation involves not only enhancing existing medical knowledge but also acquiring new skills in data science, machine learning, and bioinformatics. Physicians and healthcare providers must embrace a mindset of lifelong learning to stay abreast of these developments and their implications for patient care.

For medical professionals, a foundational understanding of AI is crucial. Doctors and nurses should seek educational opportunities that bridge the gap between clinical practice and technology. This could include workshops, online courses, or degree programs focusing on AI applications in healthcare. Understanding algorithms and data interpretation will enable healthcare providers to better utilize AI-driven diagnostic tools, enhancing their ability to deliver precise and personalized care. Additionally, engaging with interdisciplinary teams will foster a collaborative environment where medical knowledge and technical expertise converge to improve patient outcomes.

Medical researchers play a vital role in the development and validation of AI technologies. Training in data science and bioinformatics is essential for those seeking to innovate within the field. Researchers must learn to design studies that effectively integrate AI methodologies, ensuring that the results are reliable and applicable in clinical settings. This includes understanding predictive analytics, which can lead to breakthroughs in patient monitoring and treatment strategies. By equipping themselves with these skills, researchers can contribute significantly to advancements in AI-based drug discovery and the development of effective therapeutic interventions.

Healthcare administrators face the challenge of implementing AI solutions within their organizations. Training in project management, change management, and technology assessment will be key in navigating the complexities of integrating AI into existing systems. Administrators should be well-versed in the ethical considerations surrounding AI, particularly regarding patient data privacy and security. This knowledge will enable them to make informed decisions that promote the responsible and effective use of AI technologies, ensuring that healthcare institutions can harness the full potential of these innovations while maintaining trust with patients and stakeholders.

For students in computer science, engineering, and data science, aligning their education with the needs of the healthcare sector is paramount. Curricula should include specialized courses that focus on AI applications in medical imaging analysis, telemedicine solutions, and mental health support. By collaborating with healthcare professionals, students can gain insights into real-world challenges and develop practical solutions that address these issues. This interdisciplinary approach will not only prepare students for careers in healthcare technology but also foster innovation that enhances patient care through AI. As the demand for intelligent solutions in healthcare grows, a well-prepared workforce will be essential to drive the future of AI in this vital field.

Chapter 11: Conclusion

Summary of Key Insights

The integration of artificial intelligence into healthcare has ushered in a transformative era, enabling improved diagnostic accuracy and personalized treatment plans. AI-driven diagnostic tools leverage vast datasets to identify patterns that may elude human observation, ultimately enhancing clinical decision-making. By synthesizing data from various sources, including electronic health records, genetic information, and real-time patient monitoring, these tools empower healthcare professionals to deliver more precise and effective care.

Personalized medicine has gained significant traction through the application of AI technologies. By analyzing individual patient profiles, AI algorithms can recommend tailored treatment options that consider a patient's genetic makeup, lifestyle, and medical history. This shift towards personalization not only improves patient outcomes but also fosters a more efficient healthcare system by minimizing adverse effects and unnecessary interventions. The ability to customize therapies based on predictive models represents a major advancement in how healthcare providers approach treatment.

AI's role in medical imaging analysis has also seen remarkable progress, with machine learning algorithms enhancing the interpretation of imaging studies such as X-rays, MRIs, and CT scans. These advanced tools can detect anomalies with a speed and accuracy that complements radiologists' expertise, thereby reducing diagnostic errors and expediting treatment initiation. As AI continues to evolve, its applications in imaging will likely expand, further solidifying its position as a critical component of modern diagnostic processes.

Predictive analytics powered by AI is reshaping patient care strategies by enabling early intervention and more proactive management of chronic conditions. By utilizing historical patient data and real-time monitoring, AI systems can forecast potential health risks, allowing healthcare providers to implement preventive measures. This capability not only enhances patient safety but also contributes to cost savings for healthcare organizations by reducing hospital readmissions and emergency visits.

Finally, AI-enhanced telemedicine solutions are revolutionizing access to healthcare, especially in underserved areas. By facilitating remote consultations and continuous health monitoring, these technologies bridge the gap between patients and healthcare providers, ensuring that individuals receive timely support and intervention. Moreover, AI's application in mental health monitoring offers innovative approaches to understanding and managing mental health conditions, providing valuable insights that can guide treatment plans. As these advancements continue to unfold, the potential for AI to transform healthcare practices remains vast and promising.

Call to Action for Healthcare Stakeholders

Healthcare stakeholders must recognize the critical role they play in the integration of AI-driven diagnostics into modern medical practice. Doctors and physicians stand at the forefront of patient care. By embracing AI technologies, they can enhance diagnostic accuracy, streamline workflows, and ultimately improve patient outcomes. It is essential for healthcare professionals to familiarize themselves with the capabilities of these technologies, thus enabling them to leverage tools that provide insights into patient data, identify patterns in symptoms, and recommend personalized treatment plans. This shift towards AI-assisted diagnostics will not only elevate the standard of care but also empower physicians to focus more on patient interaction and less on administrative tasks.

Nurses and allied healthcare professionals also play a vital role in the adoption of AI in clinical settings. Their unique position allows them to bridge the gap between technology and patient care. By engaging with AI-driven tools, nurses can enhance their ability to monitor patient conditions in real-time, anticipate potential complications, and communicate more effectively with physicians. Training programs that focus on the use of AI technologies in nursing practice will be crucial. This will not only ensure that nurses are equipped with the necessary skills but also foster a culture of collaboration between healthcare teams and technology, ultimately leading to better patient care and outcomes.

Medical researchers and academia have a significant responsibility to advance the integration of AI in healthcare. By conducting rigorous research and trials, they can validate the effectiveness of AI-driven diagnostic tools and showcase their potential in various medical fields. Collaboration with technology developers will be essential in creating evidence-based solutions that meet the demands of healthcare providers. Additionally, researchers should focus on ethical considerations and data privacy concerns related to AI in healthcare, ensuring that innovations are not only effective but also responsible. This commitment to ethical research will encourage the adoption of AI technologies by practitioners who are often hesitant about new tools.

For students in computer science, engineering, and data science, the call to action is clear: equip yourself with the knowledge and skills to contribute to the evolving healthcare landscape. Developing AI algorithms tailored for healthcare applications, understanding data analytics, and creating user-friendly interfaces for medical practitioners are pivotal areas of focus. Engaging in interdisciplinary projects that bring together technology and healthcare will enhance their understanding of real-world applications and challenges. Students should seek internships and collaborative opportunities within healthcare settings to gain firsthand experience and insights into how AI can transform patient care.

Finally, software engineers and data scientists should prioritize the development of AI-enhanced solutions that address specific needs in healthcare. By focusing on areas such as predictive analytics for patient care, AI in medical imaging analysis, and AI-based drug discovery, they can create tools that significantly improve clinical workflows and patient outcomes. Continuous feedback from healthcare professionals will be essential in this process, ensuring that the technologies developed are user-friendly and genuinely beneficial in clinical settings. As the healthcare landscape evolves, the collaboration between technology experts and healthcare professionals will be key to harnessing the full potential of AI, ultimately leading to a more efficient, effective, and patient-centered healthcare system.

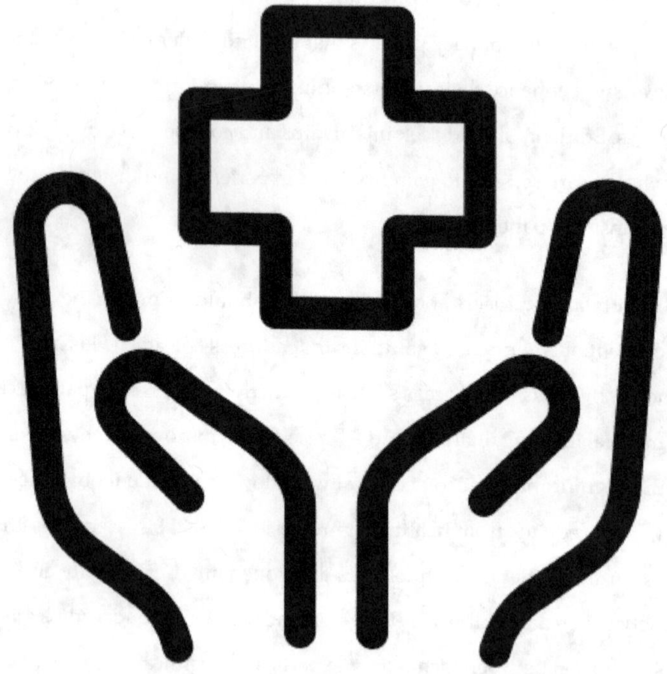

AI Heals: Revolutionizing Healthcare

Artificial Intelligence (AI) is revolutionizing the healthcare industry, promising to transform patient care and medical research. By analyzing vast amounts of data, AI-powered algorithms can detect patterns and anomalies that may be missed by human observation, leading to earlier and more accurate diagnoses. Additionally, AI can assist in drug discovery, personalize treatment plans, and optimize resource allocation.

From robotic surgery to virtual health assistants, AI is enhancing the efficiency and effectiveness of healthcare delivery. However, the integration of AI in healthcare raises ethical concerns, including data privacy, algorithmic bias, and the potential for job displacement. It is crucial to ensure that AI systems are developed and deployed responsibly, with transparency and accountability at the forefront. As AI continues to advance, it is essential to strike a balance between technological innovation and human values, prioritizing patient well-being and ethical considerations.